The

Wayward

Stork

IVF: The Wayward Stork

◆

What to expect, who to expect it from, and surviving it all…

Sarah A. Tursi, M.S.W.

Lea McCarthy

iUniverse, Inc.
New York   Lincoln   Shanghai

IVF: The Wayward Stork
What to expect, who to expect it from, and surviving it all…

Copyright © 2005 by Sarah Tursi and Lea McCarthy

iUniverse books may be ordered through booksellers or by contacting:

iUniverse
2021 Pine Lake Road, Suite 100
Lincoln, NE 68512
www.iuniverse.com
1-800-Authors (1-800-288-4677)

ISBN-13: 978-0-595-35784-0 (pbk)
ISBN-13: 978-0-595-80253-1 (ebk)
ISBN-10: 0-595-35784-9 (pbk)
ISBN-10: 0-595-80253-2 (ebk)

Printed in the United States of America

To our IVF daughters, whose difficult journey to conception inspired the creation of this book.

To our families, without their love and support the completion of this book would have remained a dream.

To all infertility patients, your strength and courage motivated us to produce a collection of emotional tools, empowering knowledge, and encouraging words to support you through your own incredible journey.

Contents

Acknowledgements

We would like to extend our endless gratitude to the fertility specialists whose genuine enthusiasm and compassion, coupled with unparalleled expertise, assisted in the making of our miracles.

Dr. William Hummel
Dr. Michael Kettel
San Diego Fertility Center

Dr. Grant W. Patton, Jr
Southeastern Fertility Center

Dr. Sherman J. Silber
The Infertility Center of Saint Louis

Our special thanks to the Obstetricians who cared for our physical and emotional well-being and who delivered our precious, long awaited little ones.

Dr. Michael DeRosa
Saint John's Hospital
"You are a great source of humor, comfort, and reassurance. I will never forget that your medical prowess saved my life. You rock!"

Dr. Margaret Marcrander
West Coast OB/GYN Associates
"You made the impossible my reality. Against the odds, you did it and I am forever grateful. She is, because you are."

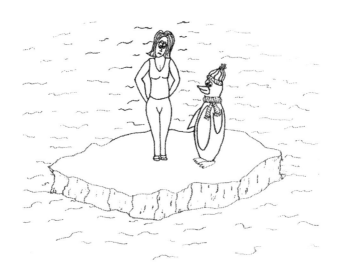

Welcome to the world of infertility; population: you. Or at least that's how we felt. We are mothers, wives, businesswomen, and infertility patients. We consider ourselves to be normal, reasonably healthy, emotionally balanced individuals who found ourselves in an extraordinary situation facing the unexpected and the unfathomable. Despite our best efforts, we are two women with infertility, which precluded us from a natural conception. We felt bewildered and lost amongst a sea of new medical terms and diagnoses. We feared the invasive tests, the injections, and the great possibility of cycle failure. We felt angry and betrayed by our bodies and the inability to do the most natural of all things! We stressed about the financial ramifications of this very expensive procedure. We felt completely and utterly alone.

We have both endured numerous miscarriages, several failed inseminations, a plethora of tests and exams, successful in vitro fertilizations (IVF), and failed frozen embryo transfers (FET).

We have sat impatiently in waiting rooms, cried tears at the pharmacy, yelled at our husbands, stuck ourselves repetitively while wiping sweaty palms and steadying shaky hands, placed all of our hopes on multiple developing follicles, urinated on those evil pee-pee tests like incontinent maniacs, and prayed for our unborn angels that God took too early.

We have laughed, we have cried, and we have thrown our French fries in the face of an unsuspecting clerk at the local fast food joint for a lack of salty goodness. Through all of the emotional chaos, we educated ourselves, we gathered adequate support, and we made a friendship with one another, which will last a lifetime.

Preface

No, it is not just you. None of us know exactly *how* we got to the point of scheduling an IVF cycle. Clearly we recall discussing with the doctors our inability to conceive or maintain a pregnancy. We were assured, in the traditional fashion, that our problems were mere "flukes." Certainly, we would get pregnant in the next few months.

"Relax."

"Don't worry!"

"Just give it some time."

"Enjoy one another before you have kids."

Those famous last words said years before reluctantly trudging to an IVF clinic. Sitting in the office waiting room, where *we* don't belong, plagued with feelings of abnormality and failure. This procedure is too extreme, an absolute last resort. All the while thinking to ourselves: "Am I really here? Did I reach the end of that line? Am I really prepared to go through with this?" We are going to be like those people you read about, those people who do really extreme things to change their reality. We have become…*those people.*

We understand how difficult it is to see this book and need it. Every needle phobic, financially draining, hormone raged aspect of it. We get it and we're here to help you though it. There is a certain disbelief that comes with entering into the world of IVF and assisted reproduction. IVF is the treatment that you read about in magazines and hear on the news. Even Oprah had special show about it! It isn't supposed to be part of *your* life.

IVF just sounds like a big deal. Medical procedures themselves are often enough to evoke feelings of fear and anxiety. For many women, the thought of the necessary injections is over-whelming. For some, a simple blood test is a huge deal, let alone intramuscular injections administered every single day for over a month!

"There is no way that *my* husband is injecting me…no way."

In addition to the injections, women fear the numerous procedures. Hysterosalpingograms (HSG), ultrasounds, frequent blood work, physical examinations…the list goes on and on. Most of the interventions are invasive. Many are described as painful. Who would sign up for this torture? Well, the thousands of women who are dying to become mothers. That's who! Women, who could never bring themselves to donate blood for fear of a needle stick, yet would cut off their right arm for a healthy baby to bring home. Women, who spend their days and nights praying for a positive pregnancy test, and the weeks to follow, depressed and heartbroken. Women…like us.

When choosing to endure an IVF cycle, every woman must confront numerous issues before committing to treatment.

"What about the risk of multiples?"

"What if I succeed and then experience a pregnancy loss?"

"What will my family think?"

"What are the social stigmas associated with IVF?"

"Am I ready to have a test tube baby?"

Maybe the bigger looming question is: "*Can* I have a test tube baby?"

For many of us, the biggest fear of all is the fear of cycle failure. Hope is what keeps us all going. There is a hope that all of the research and technology will pay off and that we, along with millions of other folks, will finally become parents.

In Vitro Fertilization

In vitro fertilization, what's that all about? Remember back to seventh grade health class when we learned that fertilization occurs during sexual intercourse when the egg and sperm meet? (tee-hee) There was a sense, even back in the day, that the process wasn't entirely mechanical. In vitro fertilization is all of the mechanics with none of the thrill. There is no zippity-do-dah happening here!

In the United States, an estimated 6.1 million couples are infertile. Fewer than 5% of infertile couples seeking treatment will participate in vitro fertilization. By the age of 19, the likelihood of an egg from a healthy woman being fertilized during unprotected sex is about 26%. By the age of 41, the chances are fewer than 5%. At birth, the average woman has one million eggs. By the age of your first period, you have approximately 300 to 400 thousand. Does it seem like the odds are against you on this one?

Simply stated, in vitro fertilization allows for an egg and a sperm to create an embryo, in a controlled environment, outside of the mother's body. First, your ovaries are hyper-stimulated, through the use of hormones, to produce multiple eggs. At maturity, your eggs are harvested and mixed with sperm in a culture dish and monitored for fertilization. Fertilized eggs are then placed into your uterus, in the hopes that one will attach to the uterine wall and develop into a fetus. Additional embryos, if any, may be frozen for later cycle attempts.

Infertility treatment is not sequential. This is not a generic staircase with IVF being the final step. In vitro fertilization should not be thought of as a last-ditch attempt at conception. There is a multitude of factors that should dictate which treatments are the most effective for you and your personal case.

Many women have wasted months, or even years, with infertility treatments that have not worked for their issues, simply because of cost or fear. In some cases, IVF may be the first step, and not the last, during infertility treatment. However you got here, you're here. And we're with you. IVF may appear overwhelming, but it is do-able.

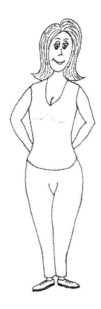

1

Preparing for Your IVF

Infertile. How can that be? We are normal, hard-working, happily married people who live the right way and make good choices. We *always* replace the toilet paper on the holder, return the grocery cart to the corral, and stop at yellow lights. So, there is obviously some mistake.

Like every woman longing to conceive, we feel this month we will get pregnant. We find ourselves thinking: "Something definitely feels different this time." Certainly, we are more tired, our boobs are sore, and we are undoubtedly urinating more frequently! Each and every symptom in the book, right? And those evil home pregnancy tests! Squinting to see a second line, holding the stick up to the light for a better view.

"I can see a line, can't you?"

Besides, the timing was *perfect*. How could we not be pregnant? We did everything right! Our personal struggles are not uncommon. From charting cycles and taking temperatures, to In uterine inseminations (IUI), the doctors say everything looks perfect. Perfect, but childless. What is going wrong?

For some of us, that positive test has yet to appear. For others, there have been numerous positive pregnancy tests without a cute, fat bundle of joy to show for it. Regardless, we convince ourselves that *this* cycle will be different. We joke with friends that infertility has become our new hobby. In all reality, it does consume our lives. All of our time and money invested into this one pursuit. Everything revolves around our cycle. Now, we are in the home stretch of technology: IVF.

We cannot stress enough that no one, truly *no one*, will be as invested in your care and a successful outcome as you. You are your own best advocate. You are your own best researcher, investigator, and records keeper. Know your medical information better than anyone treating you. This is the time to become an expert in your infertility issues. Many women come to their first IVF cycle in total bewilderment at the core "problem." Unexplained infertility is frustrating but is not an end all be all diagnosis that removes responsibility from the patient to know how her body is or is not responding during each cycle. Take your control back, girlfriend! Infertility is not something that is happening to you, it's something that is happening with you. Empower yourself with knowledge. It is tremendously important to be an educated consumer. Think about it. Would you spend $10,000 on a product that you know little about?

A good rule of thumb is "ask and document." You know more than you think about your infertility. Take the time to review your obstetrical history. You probably know what tests you have had done and when these procedures were conducted. Do some research and find out exactly what the results were. You can request your records from your primary care doctor, your OB/GYN, or other practitioners who have cared for your health. Pull together additional related events, such as the age you started your period. Construct a file of every test and appointment that you have had relating to your fertility. Make a timeline of your history. Boom! Before you know it, you've got yourself an invaluable tool to share with your doctor.

> Your chart might look something like this:
>
> Age 12—onset of menstruation
> Age 15—medical intervention for severe menstrual cramping
> Age 20—started on birth control pills
> Age 20—became sexually active
> Age 23—treated for an STD, infected partner
> Age 28—pelvic inflammatory disease diagnosed after a
>   colposcopy
> Age 29—week five miscarriage, no medical intervention

It is imperative that you maintain records of your current fertility interventions and understand how that pertains to your cycle. Make a habit of obtaining and recording all medical information as it becomes available to you. Write it down, no matter how inconsequential it may seem. When the nursing staff informs you of your lab results, document the following information:

+ What test was conducted?
+ Why was this test conducted?
+ What is the expected result?
+ What is your result?
+ What would be considered problematic?
+ How does this result relate to your cycle?
+ What is the next step?

We are all painfully aware of the negative occurrences which are possible with our cycle, but are ill informed as to how such decisions are made as a result. For example, many women fear that their IVF cycle will be cancelled due to a poor response, however they remain ignorant as to the criteria that makes cancellation necessary. There are many choices made throughout each IVF cycle. Which medications at what dosage, what point should my cycle be triggered, and when is the appropriate time for my egg retrieval? These decisions should be made with your input and thoughts behind them. Your doctor is treating tens, if not hundreds, of women. In all probability, your medical professional may not specifically remember your complete medical profile when making quick decisions about your care.

Certainly, you want to select a doctor based on his or her credentials and statistical evaluation of success. Although you should trust that you are under the best care, this intensive level of medical intervention calls for a very involved patient. Your office staff truly will welcome your questions and helpful input. For example, if you have a history of over-stimulation, your doctor will want to be reminded of that. If you have had a greater success on a specific medication, you will want to reiterate that information when your doctor is making medication decisions. IVF is a team effort. Maybe you can get a pair of scrubs out of this deal! You will receive the best of care when you and your doctor work closely together. When you are informed and involved, you will most likely be privy to more information from your doctor. This is a fantastic way to establish a more personable relationship. Avoid becoming just another patient. He or she will come to know your particular case better and thus be more invested in your outcome.

The best source of medical information will not only come from your doctor and IVF clinic, but also from the multitude of websites dedicated to the subject of IVF treatment. You will want to frequent those websites to keep updated on the latest technology and treatments available. The importance of knowing what other major IVF clinics are doing to get women pregnant is vital to aggressively seeking the best medical care available. Technology, medication, and treatments are rapidly changing. Medical books become dated before they are printed. Stay up to date with the latest interventions via the medical and IVF websites and patient chat rooms. This will help you make educated decisions about your care. Also, it will help guide you in your choice of doctors and clinics.

Choosing a Fertility Clinic

All too often, women say that the clinic chooses them, they did not specifically choose the clinic. Many of us started our IVF journey with our primary care physician or our regular OB/GYN doctor. Some women switch their care to a Reproductive Endocrinologist when they are first diagnosed with infertility. Many of the tests and procedures to diagnose infertility problems can be conducted at the OB/GYN office. Thus, many women stay with this first tier service provider.

We have a bias in writing this book: *Run*, don't walk, to a fertility specialist! Although your OB/GYN doctor may be fantastic in every way, he or she cannot give you the level of care that you now require for this particular concern. You need to be treated by a physician who has the benefit of specialized experience with similar cases as well as a familiarity with the latest medical advances in fertility medications and state of the art treatments. Experience is invaluable in this field.

Additionally, it is very important to investigate the statistical success of that particular clinic. Under the Fertility Clinic Success Rate and Certification Act, the Centers for Disease Control and Prevention (CDC) and the Society for Assisted Reproductive Technology (SART) compiles the type, number, and outcome of ART cycles performed in U.S. clinics into yearly reports.

Fertility clinics are compared by the following criteria:
+ Number of IVF transfers performed
+ Number of pregnancies achieved
+ Number of actual live births
+ Number of multiple births
+ Age of the IVF patient

This information also includes which clinics are reporting their statistics and which are not. The InterNational Council on Infertility Information Dissemination (INCIID, pronounced as "inside") is a wonderful source of information on clinics and offers a list of member providers.

Do not be fooled! Not all IVF clinics are equal. Typically, the best clinics perform a lot of IVF procedures annually. The incidence of multiple births should be lower than other facilities. The larger IVF clinics generally have good funding, and are able to court the very best doctors, researchers, and embryologists in the industry. Often times, these doctors have published books or articles on infertility or specific fertility treatments. The cost of treatment will vary from clinic to clinic. Do not make the assumption that the larger, better known clinics will be more expensive. Often times, the opposite is true. Do not be afraid to contact that world famous physician for your IVF treatment. They, too, treat individual patients and may take your case. You can always benefit from cutting edge research and technology. After all, the ultimate goal is to become pregnant and deliver a healthy baby.

It is very important to select a clinic that can provide you a broad range of treatments and procedures. Frequently, women will talk about the need to switch doctors or facilities because they cannot get the level of treatment they may require to achieve pregnancy. Make certain that your doctor and associated clinic can provide all of the diagnostic and treatment options that may be applicable to your situation. Make sure you understand who specifically will be treating you, both during the diagnostic period, as well as throughout your IVF cycle. Know how long that doctor will handle your care, if and when you become pregnant. It is imperative that you are able to effectively communicate with your Reproductive Endocrinologist, the embryologist, the hospital lab, and your OB/GYN.

Be an educated consumer. IVF is a business. Unlike other areas of medicine, there is a profit being made directly from the patient. Some fortunate few may have partial or full insurance coverage. However, most women end up paying for half or more of their IVF treatment out of pocket.

The following are some survival tips to help guide you in choosing the clinic that is right for you:

+ Ask for a referral from your trusted OB/GYN or general practitioner.

+ Call other OB/GYN offices and inquire as to where they refer their patients.

+ Look for a center that has performed hundreds or thousands of IVF cycles. Experience is the key here. The more cycles performed, the more experience and knowledge is gained as a result.

+ Interview the Reproductive Endocrinologist and the embryologist, if possible, of all potential clinics to get a feel of their expertise, confidence, and the most up-to-date techniques they offer. Assess your personality compatibility with the primary fertility specialist. Will your concerns be given the appropriate merit? Will you be viewed as a partner in this process? Compare your findings from all available clinics.

+ Don't be put off by traveling to a clinic. Many experienced clinics are prepared to handle out-of-town patients. Limiting yourself to your local IVF clinic may prove to be detrimental in the long run.

+ Ask them for a list of former patients who may be willing to give you a first-hand account of the benefits and downfalls of that potential clinic.

+ Learn everything you can about the fertility center you are considering. Take a tour, meet the nurses, investigate the examination and procedure rooms, and familiarize yourself with the office policies regarding test results, appointments, and after-hours emergencies.

> ✦ IVF is a money-making business, treat it as such. Your clinic is sure to!
>
> ✦ Trust your instincts.

Maximizing Your Benefits

Now is the time to locate and review that huge insurance coverage booklet you received when you, or your spouse, signed up for your current health insurance plan. Read, and reread, the sections in your book that pertain to covered benefits for maternity and infertility treatments. Make two photocopies of that specific page and submit one copy to your clinic or hospital's billing office and keep the other on your person. Additionally, it is very helpful to have several copies of your insurance card, both front and back, along with that coverage page. It is also advised to make copies of any paper referrals that you have been given and of all prescriptions as well.

You must know exactly what is covered by your insurance plan and what your out-of-pocket expenses will be. Often, people pay more than their required share due to policy coverage and benefit ignorance. If you find the language difficult to understand, call the insurance company directly for clarification. Note the time and the date of your phone call, as well as the name of the representative you spoke with and the information obtained. Many times, your hospital or clinic can process your prescriptions or lab requests through your primary care or OB/GYN physician for additional benefit coverage. It is important to know what referrals you must have in place in order to take full advantage of your coverage. It is possible to have prescriptions written to accommodate multiple blood draws, ultrasounds, or medication refills.

Some insurance companies require that you participate in their infertility program. You may be given a specific phone number to call with questions or needs. Additionally, you may be assigned a specific care manager to help you through the insurance issues. Let them help you! They can walk you through the insurance maze, making certain that you are tapping into your full coverage potential. Get educated, be prepared, and utilize all that is available to you.

Financially Speaking

It can be overwhelming to critically examine the cost of financing an IVF cycle. It would be more fun to indulge in a 'round the world adventure, perhaps own a luxury vehicle, or even get some much needed liposuction! While our friends talk of kitchen renovations and expensive jewelry, we are forced to cough up our life savings for medication, lab work, and ultrasounds. No, it's not fair. Having a baby should be fun. A romp in the hay, followed by an exciting announcement over a fantastic meal.

Hopefully, *your* exciting announcement is just down the road a bit. The costs of your IVF cycle is in the here and now. It is appropriate to request an estimated total cost of your IVF cycle from your clinic. They should have a prepared overview of all expected expenses and an approximate payment timetable. Understand the costs associated with individual medications, lab work, procedures, and possible hospital admissions. It is smart to comparison shop when looking for a pharmacy. Medication prices vary greatly, so check into various specialty pharmacies, both local and online. Ask your clinic for referrals to local and national pharmacies.

Your physician may offer a patient medication share program. Many clinics allow patients to donate leftover medication after a successful treatment cycle or when the treatment protocol has evolved to include a new medication. Some clinics receive samples of medications that they are willing to share with patients without insurance coverage. Don't be afraid to ask! Being proactive and inquisitive can save you thousands of dollars.

Once you are aware of all of the costs involved with IVF, you can then assess how to best finance your treatment. There are numerous resources for financing an IVF cycle. Speak to the financial specialist at your clinic and do some independent research online.

Some clinics have a guarantee program, commonly referred to as "Shared Risk", where you can pay one flat rate for three IVF cycles. You will recover a specified portion of that money if you do not become pregnant within those three cycles. However, if you become pregnant on your first cycle, you will have most likely overpaid and will not see a refund for the difference. For some couples, this is a great way of putting a ceiling on the money allotted to IVF treatments. Many people feel that they will either be successful in having a child and therefore it will be well worth the total investment or that they will recover some funds which could then be applied to additional treatments or possibly adoption.

There is, however, a catch. The companies that sponsor these "Shared Risk" insurance policies will investigate your "appropriateness" for their program, based on age, diagnosis, pre-existing medical conditions, and other such criteria. Simply put: you will either be turned down entirely or accepted because you are most likely to conceive before three IVF attempts. It is important when considering these programs to talk with your doctor about your personal, statistical likelihood of conception and live birth. Know what your chances are and into which category you fall. Explore all of your financial options and keep an open mind.

Managing Work

For most of us, there is a huge balancing act between work and our personal life. It is very difficult to maintain privacy about IVF when alter you work schedule due to cycle appointments. You may decide to discuss your IVF with your boss or supervisor so that they are aware of why you require so much flexibility during this time. Be honest about the fact that there is no way to accurately predict when you will need to be out for an appointment. There is very little flexibility with this treatment. Highlight the 10 to 12 days of your stimulation phase and offer the estimated date of retrieval. You will be going to blood draws and ultrasounds at least every other day for this period of time.

Most clinics require morning appointments. You may be able to schedule appointments prior to the start of your workday. Allow for extra time. This is the busiest time for clinics and the longest waits occur in the morning. Every afternoon, following ultrasounds and blood work appointments, you will be receiving instructional phone calls from your clinic. The nurse will go over the results of your tests and give you the plan for medication. Determine where and when you will be available for these phone calls. If you plan on phoning your clinic for instructions, prearrange that with your clinic staff. They may be able to target times that they generally telephone patients so that you can make yourself available.

To maintain your sanity during the work week, keep quick breakfast foods, extra panty hose, makeup, hairbrush, and a cell phone charger in your desk. The mornings will be hectic for this period of time. You will find that you forget a lot of routine information. Your normal daily schedule goes out the window. Any convenience that can be anticipated, should be anticipated.

Many women find that they are forced to miss a lot of morning work time during this stage of IVF treatment. The required tests do not mandate a full, or even half day, off of work, yet they cut into the workday frequently. You may be able to negotiate banking some overtime prior to your stimulation phase. Even a few hours of overtime can make you feel better about missing hours on several consecutive days. Business trips are not going to be possible during this time.

Set firm limits on what you are unwilling and unable to do. Now is not the time to plan and execute a large meeting or a vital presentation. Although not as fun as a trip to Hawaii, consider cashing in some of your vacation time for your cycle. This may significantly reduce your stress level. Honestly evaluate your physical and emotional needs and how consuming this process is. Prioritize your life and work.

Emotional Preparation

You are venturing into the unfamiliar. This is new to you and your partner. Maybe this will get you pregnant! You are learning a lot about your personal strengths and ability to confront tough issues head on. Hope is your motivation. It will give you the strength to jab that needle into your leg, to hear the test results and make tough decision, and to feel positive when your body feels wrecked. Get excited about the new treatment, technology, and expertise that has become available to you.

As you contemplate your upcoming IVF, decide which support people you want to bring on this journey with you. You may have a wealth of people in your life that know about your infertility struggles or you may have kept this information very private. You must decide how you want to handle this passage in your life. Gather the support from the people around you.

That support can come in a variety of different ways. You may have friends that will be interested in every detail of your treatment. They may be counted on for daily phone conversations and will appreciate updates on every lab test result. There may be friends that are helpful because they are not intrusive. Those individuals are a good source of entertainment or conversation having nothing to do with infertility or your cycle. They are simply fun and easy to be around. Perhaps there are family members that are aware of your pending IVF. You may want to enlist their help in the upcoming months. Sometimes, simply having dinner plans feels supportive.

Share your IVF calendar with a very select few. Evaluate your friends and family and chose those who are most accepting and supportive of you and your choices. Identify the most emotionally stable and strong people from your support system. Trust them with the specifics, like what days and times things are happening. Ask them to respect your decision to refrain from releasing details to all of the other important people in your life. Although many people may know that you are undergoing IVF treatment, only your select few should be aware of the day you will get the ultimate results of this cycle. Let these folks in your inner circle know that they are your only support system during this difficult time.

This is an ever-changing and difficult process with numerous daily ups and downs. The last thing you need is a well meaning, yet ignorant, friend to ask you if you are pregnant, while you are still struggling with the stress of embryo quality, cell division, and fertilization rates. Keep these people in the dark and utilize their friendship to cheer you up during difficult days or to keep you entertained during the dreaded two-week wait.

Now is not the time to resurrect a friendship. As much as we love our friends and family, please use caution when counting on certain individuals to "rise to the occasion." Keep in mind: once a selfish pain in the neck, always a selfish pain in the neck. Put your faith and trust in people who have proven dependable, predictable, and loyal. This is a very personal and emotional journey. Chose your travel mates wisely. Should you encounter those well meaning but misguided individuals, it is acceptable to remind them of the following:

- ✦ Please do not suggest that I give up on my dream of having a child until I am ready. I need this process and am fully aware of adoption and other options.

- ✦ Do not tell me that I should just be happy if I already have a child. This is not a fix for my desire for more children or a sibling for my child. I need to be afforded the same right to want this as any other woman.

- ✦ Please do not comment on my change in appearance. I understand that I look tired and maybe I have gained a pound or two. I am undergoing a major medical event, that's just par for the course.

Many women opt to get their emotional fortification from a trained, licensed therapist who specializes in infertility. Your doctor, clinic, or insurance company can help you find a professional in your area. There is something to be said for having someone outside of your inner circle to talk to. This way, you don't have to factor anyone else's feelings into the conversation. Therapy is all about you and your agenda. Sometimes that feels great!

Another fantastic resource for support is the multitude of websites with chat rooms for women going through IVF. It may be helpful to talk to people who are going through the same experiences, emotions, medications, and procedures as you. You can learn a lot of insider tips and accumulate pertinent questions to ask your doctor. Generally, the women on these sites are very well versed on the issues of infertility and IVF. They will gladly share all that they know. There are several website chats that will link you with women who are cycling with IVF at the same time.

Consider joining a local chapter of RESOLVE National Infertility Association. Multiple support groups for women going through infertility and IVF treatments are available. Additionally, they offer a plethora of information ranging from assisted reproduction to adoption and everything in between. They have a wealth of published resources, as well as organized conferences pertaining to infertility. Most major cities have local RESOLVE chapters and they are also available online.

Use this time to gather your emotional resources. The most important thing is to circle your wagons in a way that is best for you. Just focus on getting the support that you need to make it through your IVF intact.

Physical Preparation

There is so much to consider while undergoing IVF treatment. You must be aware of how your treatment affects your body and how your body affects the treatment. Now is a great time to look at your physical self and determine what behaviors or habits you want to change that could possibly increase your chances of having a successful outcome.

Many women schedule a preconception appointment with their OB/GYN. It is a good time for an annual physical and a baseline PAP smear, as well as a breast exam. A visit to the dentist isn't a bad idea either. If dental care evokes anxiety, you will not want to schedule an appointment in the middle of a pregnancy, as most medication will not be available to you. Additionally, if you whiten your teeth, this may be your last month to do so until after you deliver. The same goes for having your hair straightened or relaxed. If you have considered losing some extra weight, the months prior to your would cycle would be the time to do it. Many doctors feel that obtaining a healthy weight is vital for achieving pregnancy. Even if the goal isn't weight loss, exercise can be a wonderful stress reliever during this waiting period. As can a fantasizing about the pool boy, eating a Ho-Ho, or getting your toenails painted! Be sure to ask your doctor about restrictions on exercise during treatment. Some clinics may not want women to exercise or alter their metabolism in any way during the IVF cycle.

Because you are investing about six weeks of your life, significant sums of money, and all of your hopes and dreams into this IVF treatment, consider eliminating any unhealthy habits that could decrease your chances of conception. Drinking alcohol and smoking are two obvious behaviors of concern for both you and your partner. Additionally, you may want to eliminate caffeine and artificial sweeteners from your diet. Many doctors believe there is a connection between these substances and a failure to conceive. It stands to reason that the healthier you can be, the better your odds of conception are. Take this time to be empowered and proactive. So often in fertility treatment, there is very little we can do to create a successful outcome. Do everything you can to make it happen!

There are two things that you can do to significantly impact your cycle outcome. The first is to take prenatal vitamins as prescribed. This is one of the few "no brainers" in fertility treatment. Give your body every opportunity to conceive by having enough folic acid and B vitamins onboard. The second is to ensure that you are consuming plenty of protein during this time. Additional protein will not only give you a lasting feeling of being full, but it is a natural way of managing your stress level. Sugars can make women feel sluggish, irritable, and anxious. Protein will serve as a natural absorber of excess adrenaline thus making you more likely to feel calm and in control.

Commonly, it is suggested to reduce your stress before and during IVF. *Isn't that the most ridiculous thought!* We are embarking on the most frustrating, expensive, scary, and helpless adventure that life has thrown so far, but *reduce your stress?* I'll get right on that! It is in the same vein as "relax, drink some wine, go on vacation and you will get pregnant." Understandably, you are stressed. Additionally, you may be worried, preoccupied, and absolutely disgusted beyond belief. For the purposes of this book, we will say that the goal is to *manage* your stress.

You can use this time as an opportunity to prioritize the activities in your schedule and how you commit to those activities. Maybe this is the time in your life that you prioritize *you* first. Give yourself permission to set limits in your life, work, and relationships. Attempt to eliminate some of the "have to's". You may not feel like attending your mother-in-law's family dinner, or attending a girl's night out, or making an appearance at the work-sponsored picnic. Even if others do not understand, distance yourself from other obligations to allow for time to recoup, both physically and emotionally, from injections, test results, appointments, and procedures. This is your time. Use it to pamper yourself and focus on your own personal needs.

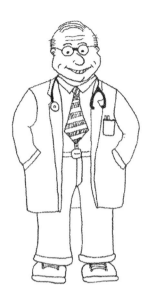

2

Pre-IVF Testing

Before your IVF cycle can begin, your doctor may order a plethora of tests. Hold on to your hat, there are an awful lot of hoops to jump through. Many clinics require that you undergo at least baseline blood work, day three labs, a preparation cycle, a mock transfer, a Hysterosalpinogram (HSG), and a clearing ultrasound. Typically, a recent semen analysis and blood work from your partner is also a requirement. Although these tests may seem inconvenient, they provide your doctor with valuable information that can greatly impact your chances of conception. Your doctor may order additional testing as needed. If you have recently completed some of these tests through your primary care physician or OB/GYN, it is perfectly appropriate to ask if it is possible to avoid retesting.

Most of us feel a sense of urgency and a desire to move on to the treatment cycle as quickly as possible. After all, you wanted that baby yesterday, right? Ask your clinic how many tests you can get done within the same cycle. You can also request the month you are scheduled for your IVF. Having a specified date to look forward to can help ease the waiting time.

Preparation Cycle

A preparation cycle may be recommended by your doctor to determine how your body will respond to various medications. Although you may feel like you are sitting on "Go", it can be useful to have a warm-up cycle in order for your physician to know how to gauge your medication levels. Some women will hyper-stimulate on a moderate amount of medication, which may then result in their cycle being cancelled. Others will not be stimulated enough and a poor response will result in a cancelled cycle, as well. Unless you have endured other follicle stimulating hormone (FSH) medicated cycles, your doctor may determine that this information is necessary to reduce the chance of cycle cancellation.

Baseline Blood Work

These blood tests can be administered at any point in your cycle. Often times, your doctor will order this blood work at your initial appointment.

Your baseline blood work may include some of the following tests:

+ Complete Blood Count (CBC)
+ Thyroid Function
+ HIV Screening
+ Chemistry Profile
+ Hepatitis B
+ Hepatitis C
+ Blood Type
+ Rh Factor
+ Rubella
+ Hormonal Analysis

Day Three Blood Work

On cycle day three, your doctor will order a blood draw to examine the FSH and estradiol (E2) hormone levels present in your system. FSH stimulates the development of ovarian follicles. An FSH level under 10 on cycle day three is considered favorable. A high FSH or E2 on cycle day three is an indication of decreased ovarian reserve, meaning your egg supply is limited. The information collected from your day three blood work will give your doctor a good indication of your expected stimulation response. Women with decreased ovarian reserve are typically poor responders to fertility drugs. These lab results will help determine the most appropriate dosage of fertility medication necessary to initiate proper ovarian stimulation. Ask your doctor to explain your individual day three values and what it means for your fertility.

Trial Transfer

Similar to a practice drill, many clinics will perform a trial transfer, or mock embryo transfer. This serves as a practice run for your doctor and assisting nurses. Although nothing is being injected and no embryos are transferred, detailed notes are taken during the procedure, which will be helpful to your doctor during the actual event. Your doctor may describe this procedure as similar to a PAP smear. You will be asked to place your feet in stirrups. With the aide of a speculum, a small catheter will be placed through your cervix. The cervix is very similar to a sphincter, the more you clench, the tighter it gets. Do yourself a favor and relax. Employ all relaxation techniques, such as deep breathing and visualization. Many women describe this procedure as uncomfortable. However, this should not be ranked on your top ten most painful list. If you find yourself particularly uncomfortable, you can ask for a mild sedative during this procedure.

Ultrasound

It is important to note that all ultrasounds for IVF are transvaginal, meaning that they are performed through the vagina instead of on the surface of the lower abdomen. There is no need to drink a lot of water, which is a huge relief to women with sensitive bladders! You may be more comfortable emptying your bladder prior to the ultrasound. You can eat and drink normally prior to this procedure. It can be helpful to wear "easy on/easy off" clothing. Removing panty hose and attempting to put them back on in a tiny dressing room or bathroom is a huge pain in the neck. The technician will give you a paper sheet to wrap your lower half in. You can, and should, stay dressed from the waist up. Wearing a longer shirt may allow you to preserve the sanctity of your smiling backside. The less than adequate paper sheet will not conceal your fandoonie.

During the ultrasound, you will lie back on the examination table and place your feet in stirrups. You may be asked to place the probe into your vagina. The ultrasound tech will measure your uterine lining and ensure that your ovaries are quiet and ready for stimulation.

Hysterosalpinogram (HSG)

This very common test is used to examine the condition of your uterus and fallopian tubes. An HSG takes about one hour to perform. You will be asked to lie on your back similar to a PAP smear, under an X-ray. Radio-opaque dye will be passed in a catheter through your cervix and into your uterus. Uterine abnormalities, such as unusual shape, tumors, or scar tissue, which may prevent embryo implantation, can be seen on the X-ray. The dye is expected to flow through the fallopian tubes, allowing the radiologist to visualize any blockages. If your tubes are open, the dye will fill and illuminate your tubes on the X-ray. If you have a blockage, the dye will not pass. This provides your doctor with valuable information about the health and functionality of your tubes and uterus.

Your HSG will be performed between cycle day six and eleven. If you are required to have this test done, make certain to schedule it as soon as possible to avoid a frustrating month-long delay. You are likely to be advised that this test is only mildly uncomfortable. Some doctors are prone to hopeless min-imalization. Ladies, don't fall victim! Some women report that this test is extremely painful and memorable years after the experience. Others are only mildly uncomfortable. Most likely, your doctor will suggest that you take a dose of over-the-counter pain medication prior to your test to minimize pain or cramping. It is appropriate and recommended that you also request a dose of Valium to relax your uterus and to alleviate the pain from associated cramping. The use of these medications is not required. However, it is the only way to assure yourself that you will not experience hair-curling pain. Additionally, you will be prescribed an antibiotic to protect your body from bacterial infections. Make certain that you take all of the medication pre-scribed to you. A resulting infection, such as pelvic inflamma-tory disease (PID), can further complicate fertility issues.

The dye used in this procedure contains iodine and is not appropriate for women who have any sensitivity. Make certain that your doctor is aware of any allergies to shellfish or iodine. There is an alternate test, a Sonohystergram, which uses a saline solution during an ultrasound exam. This should be considered for anyone who is at risk for iodine related issues.

You may not feel like going back to work after this proce-dure. Many clinics require that someone accompany you to the test and drive you home afterwards. You could feel crampy and sore for several hours after the test is completed. But the infor-mation collected from this procedure can save you time and money with inappropriate fertility treatments.

Hysteroscopy

If uterine abnormalities are discovered after the HSG, your doctor may order a hysteroscopy. A thin telescope mounted with a fiber optic light, called a hysteroscope, is inserted through the cervix into the uterus. This allows pictures to be taken of the uterus for a more accurate diagnosis. Ask you doctor to explain what you can expect from this procedure and how best to prepare.

Semen Analysis

It is only fitting that your spouse has a physical opportunity to share in the baby-making endeavor. The ultimate humiliation for every IVF husband is the dreaded semen analysis. Keep in mind that 40% of infertility is as a result of a male factor, so this test is a necessary evil. Clinics will use this sample to observe and document sperm count, percentage of motility (movement in a straight line), morphology (structural appearance), and semen volume and consistency. The only way that this can be investigated is by collecting a fresh sperm sample.

Some clinics may allow your husband to produce a sample at home in a sterile cup and then transport it to the lab for testing. If this collection method is used, your spouse must keep his sample at body temperature. This can be accomplished by keeping the cup between his legs while driving to the clinic. Typically, the sample must be returned to the clinic within an hour of collection. If your husband is afforded the luxury of an at home collection, he can to thank his lucky stars! This is not the norm.

Many clinics insist on a fresh sperm sample produced on site. Your husband will be given a cup and the introduction to *the room*. This may be a secluded treatment room that is specifically geared for the gentlemen who need a private space. Often, there are pornographic magazines and films available to assist in the collection process. It is important to note that you will not be welcomed into the collection process with your husband. Most clinics do not allow the buddy system, so expect the semen collection to be a quick, non-intimate process.

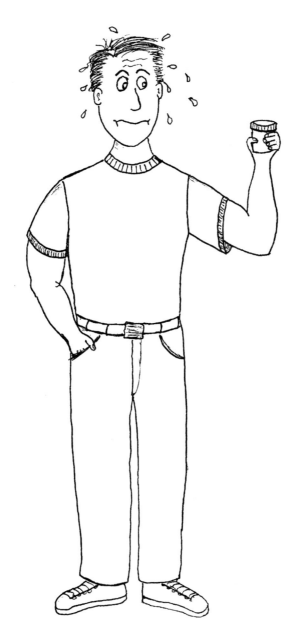

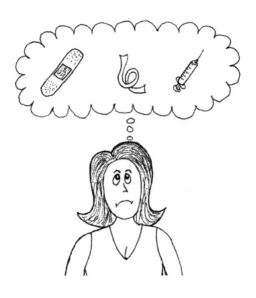

3

Tourniquets, Needles, and Band-aids, Oh My!

For many of us, injections are the most traumatic and fearfully anticipated aspect of an IVF treatment. As a general rule, we are not the gals who give blood every year, even if there are free cookies involved! Although you may not be an admitted needle-phobe, you most likely prefer to remain needle-free in your every day life.

For some, the required injections can be a deal breaker. It doesn't have to be that dramatic. There are tried and true methods that will help get you through this aspect of your treatment. You are not alone in your fear. However, you would be sadly misguided if you allowed your fear to prevent you from proceeding with IVF. Talk to your doctor about your fears. He or she is equipped to help you and your spouse meet these concerns head on.

Blood Draws

Although nobody wants to endure this, there are many ways you can help alleviate the stress and aggravation that comes with the territory. On the days that you must undergo a blood draw, wear a short-sleeved shirt for the pressure band. It is important to stay well hydrated to ensure that your veins pop out for an easier needle stick. If you have a great vein or an arm preference, express that to your nurse. Anyone can become faint on an empty stomach, so be sure to eat something before you go. Avoid pushing down on the vein after the draw, as this may increase the likelihood of bruising. Always remember that you can refuse a bandage or tape if you dislike ripping out sensitive arm hairs. Check to make sure that you have completely stopped bleeding before pulling down your sleeve or slipping on your coat. Many shirts have been ruined due to a premature rush out the door. It's always a good idea to check that your vials of blood are marked with your name and the proper test. It can be very frustrating to make a return visit to the lab as a result of an error.

Injections

Subcutaneous and intramuscular are varying types of injections to familiarize yourself with. Subcutaneous injections, or sub-Q injections, can be self-administered. The needle is short and very fine, similar to an insulin needle. Injection sites include the thigh, upper arm, or stomach, as recommended by your doctor or dictated by comfort.

Intramuscular injections, or IM injections, are most commonly administered by a nurse or spouse, if you are so trusting! For most IVF patients, having a spouse, partner, or good friend trained in administering these injections proves invaluable. Most IVF clinics will offer training to their patients prior to the start of an IVF cycle.

To alleviate some of the pain and stress of these injections, we recommend trying some of the following injection tips. (Note that these do not include drinking heavily, crying hysterically, or throwing a mini temper tantrum while chasing your spouse around the house with a needle in hand.) Remember that not all suggestions will be appropriate for your situation and you should do some personal experimenting to find what works best for you.

+ Have all of your injection materials available and organized prior to the start of the IVF cycle. Cotton balls, alcohol swabs, and sharps containers need to be at the ready.

+ You, or your injector, can practice on an orange or a styrofoam cup prior to your first injection. These surfaces mimic the resistance met by the needle in your injection site.

+ Practice, practice, practice drawing, mixing, and handling the needles. It will make the whole process much easier on you and your spouse.

+ Always check the needle prior to injection. Some needles can have flaws or "spurs" at the end that can make a needle dull and difficult to insert.

- Ask your nurse to circle each hip area with a permanent marker to identify the best site for IM injections.

- Demand a prescription of EMLA or a topical numbing cream to be used prior to the injection. Cover the numbing agent with an adhesive plastic wrap, such as Glad Press and Seal, and leave in place for at least 1 hour. The cream will greatly alleviate a majority of the localized pain. Prior to the injection, wipe off the cream, swab with the alcohol wipe, and let it dry completely. EMLA rocks! Seriously.

- Your spouse will likely be very hesitant to cause you discomfort. He may feel awful at not being able to share the burden. (However, he still may not allow you to inject him in an effort to share in the pain.) These feelings may inhibit his ability to inject you properly. Please give him permission to inject you quickly and firmly, similar to throwing a dart. Slow administration of an IM shot is more painful. Assure your partner that this pain is a temporary necessity for the conception of your baby soon-to-be.

- When receiving an IM injection, lie down on one side, bending the leg of the hip being injected. This will reduce tension in the muscle making the injection easier to administer (and receive!).

- Have a paper towel or soft tissue available for blotting the injection site after administration. Avoid using the alcohol swab as the alcohol may further irritate the injection site.

- An ice pack placed on the site, prior to the injection, may also help reduce the pain.

- Flicking the site several times or applying direct pressure to the site for one minute prior to the injection may help numb the area by confusing the nerves.

- ✦ Breath slowly and deeply in your nose and out your mouth to help your body relax. Relaxation may result in less pain.

- ✦ If you find one side of your hip is less painful to inject, continue to inject that site until it becomes sore. You are not required to alternate sides.

- ✦ Have a back up plan in the event that your spouse, or other injector, is not available. Know what your other options are. Friends in the medical field, after-hours clinics in your area, or a home health nurse are other alternatives. Your clinic may be able to make suggestions or offer additional resources.

- ✦ It is essential for you to plan your injection for the same time every day, within a 30 minute window.

PIO Injections

The progesterone in oil injection, aka: the PIO shot, has an earned reputation of being difficult by even the toughest of patients. Think of chewing Milk Duds with braces on. You can do it but it is memorably uncomfortable. Imagine hot leather seats on a 90 degree day in a bikini bottom. Do-able, but not pleasant.

Unlike medications that are dissolved in liquid, this hormone is suspended in oil. The mixture is thick and difficult to inject. Many women find that the injection site burns and becomes lumpy after the injection. You will grow to strongly dislike these shots. The administration of this IM injection typically begins after your retrieval and continues until either a negative beta test or the completion of your first trimester. Even if you possess a large posterior, you will run out of fresh injection sites. This may be the first time in your marriage that your husband will grow weary of looking at your naked behind!

Thankfully, there are fantastic ways to substantially improve your experience.

+ Warming the vial prior to the injection will liquefy the oil and expedite the injection time. You can do this by holding the vial in your hand, running it under warm water, or placing the vial in your bra.

+ Massaging the injection site will help dissipate the oil in your muscle.

+ Apply a heat source to the area before and after the injection to allow for better absorption of the oil and to ease discomfort.

+ Visually entertain yourself during the injection with a television show, a magazine, or by playing a computer game.

+ Physically distract yourself by scratching your head, wringing your hands, or talking on the phone.

+ If you find these injections to be particularly painful, speak to your doctor about switching to a different oil. Some women find that cotton seed oil is lighter than the alternatives, and results in easier administration.

+ If the penetration of the needle is painful, try a higher gauge needle. If the administration of the medication is difficult, consider a lower gauge needle. Remember, the higher the gauge, the thinner the needle. Thick oil will pass through a thinner needle at a slower rate of speed. Let your comfort dictate your needle size.

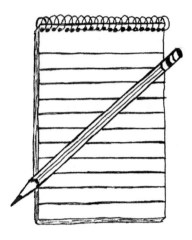

4

Beginning Your Cycle

Whew!!! Here you go. You are at the month in treatment that you have been waiting for. You may be feeling scared, excited, and overwhelmed. It is strange to have something so significant happening in your life while you are still going to work and participating in your normal routine. For the world around you, it is business as usual.

One of the most difficult aspects of IVF is fear of the unknown. It is hard to prepare for something that you may have only read about in medical terms. Our goal for this chapter is to help you navigate this journey with the advice of women who have survived. The way in which you approach treatment makes the experience manageable. Be organized and take control of what is happening in your life.

Be Prepared

Now that you are gearing up for the big game, it is important to familiarize yourself with your clinic's office policies and procedures. It is helpful to know what to expect and from whom. This will save you a lot of time on the phone and anguish when you feel like you can't wait another second for test results or for the office to open. The name of this game is "Be Prepared." There should be no surprises in what to expect from your clinic of choice.

We have compiled a list of helpful questions to ask the office staff:

- What are the office hours?
- Who answers the phone?
- How do you get your lab results?
- What if you have a medical question or concern?
- What is the after hours policy?
- How are emergencies handled?
- What specialty pharmacies do they recommend?
- Do you have a cycle coordinator who will know your individual case?
- Will they provide you with a personal treatment calendar?
- What if your procedure falls on a holiday?

Take Note

Streamline as much of your treatment as possible. Because there are so many details to remember during your IVF cycle, it is vital to create and maintain a notebook solely dedicated to this endeavor. Bring it with you to every appointment and have it ready during each phone call. This notebook will act as your IVF command center. Have a calendar of your entire treatment cycle. The date and time of every blood draw, ultrasound, and doctor appointment should be available at a glance. Write down the date and time of every injection. You do not want to schedule an evening at the theatre the night you have to begin your IM shots! Have a list of all of your contact numbers: clinic, pharmacy, lab, insurance company, therapist, and the local pizza delivery. Program the numbers that you will utilize frequently during your treatment into your cell phone for convenience. Don't rely on your memory during this month. You will temporarily lose your mind!

Your notebook should include both a copy of your insurance card and pertinent pages from your insurance coverage booklet as billing mistakes can occur easily in the midst of your treatment. Nothing is more irritating and time consuming than sorting out problems in the middle of your cycle. Knowing your insurance coverage and contact information can prevent these billing disasters from occurring. Make sure that you document if you need specific referrals for insurance coverage. Many primary care offices will not do same-day referrals. Have available all the necessary fax and phone numbers to prevent any needless running around.

Document all of the medication that you will be taking. It is very important to know when you are scheduled to take medication and at what dose. You will want to go over this medication instruction with your clinic *every* time that you speak with them. You cannot be too careful about your medication instructions. Check, and double check, all of the details about mixing medication and the timing of injections. You need to be certain that you understand the directive exactly as it is given. It is very easy to become confused about medication, dosing, mixing, and the timing of injections. Always clarify your clinic's instructions to discontinue or change medication dosage mid-cycle.

This month, you will have more blood tests than you ever thought possible. You will become an expert on which arm renders the best vein and what gauge of needle works the best for you. In this blur of tests, you will want to document every lab result. Nearing the time of your egg retrieval, you will likely undergo frequent ultrasounds to track your follicular development. Log all of the information regarding follicle size and location. These numbers, along with your lab results, will give you a better indication of how your IVF cycle is progressing. You can then prepare to be either cautiously optimistic or statistically realistic.

There is so much information thrown at you in a small period of time. You will have dozens of questions pop up throughout the month. Keep a list of these questions in your notebook and have it available for the next conversation with your doctor or nurse. These professionals are there to help you understand your cycle and the anticipated outcome. Everyone feels overwhelmed during this time. You are experiencing a huge learning curve. Do not hesitate to call the office anytime you need more information!

The ART of Survival

Your head is swimming with terminology, test results, and anticipation. To the outside world it is just another day, week, or month. To you, it's everything. Allow yourself to take a vacation from responsibilities and obligations that are optional.

So many things are completely out of your control and are simply up to luck. However, there are things that you can do to give your body the best chance of conception.

+ **Be good to yourself:** Schedule a weekly massage appointment or take a yoga class. If money is tight (duh…), take a warm bath with candles or steal a moment alone with a cup of tea. *Or* treat yourself to a Twinkie, read a trashy novel, or get hooked on the latest TV reality series. This month is no fun. Do something that you enjoy that you might typically deny yourself otherwise. This is your turn! Give yourself a little thrill to keep you going.

+ **Rest, rest, rest:** Your body is on overdrive and you need to take that into consideration. Extra sleep at night, a few naps during the day, add to your sleep bank whenever you get the chance. Remember, with a little luck, you'll have a very tiring nine months ahead. Get your sleep while you can.

+ **Entertainment:** Bring a crossword puzzle, book, or magazine to your appointments. You will spend a lot of time sitting around in waiting and exam rooms. A hand-held game system or a laptop computer can also help pass the time. Don't forget your patience, you will need it.

+ **Wear some comfortable clothing** without a restrictive waistband. You will likely become increasingly more uncomfortable as your ovaries are stimulated and the follicles grow. Make room for that expanding and tender tummy. Now's the time to pull out those comfy sweats and raid your husband's closet.

+ **Household chores:** Fill your tank with gas, have your toll money ready, stock your refrigerator, and pay your bills ahead of time. You will not want to be bothered by everyday tasks. Buy food or snacks that you can store at your office or in your car. This will make that early morning rush more manageable.

+ **Bank some overtime:** You will have to take off a lot of morning time for blood draws and ultrasounds during to your 10–12 day stimulation phase. The very start of your cycle is a good time to work a little extra. You will be glad that you did when you are running late three days in a row due to tests!

+ **Financial obligations:** Purchase gifts, cards, or schedule routine maintenance appointments now. You will not have the time, interest or memory to think of these things later in your cycle.

How To Instruct Your Inner Circle

Often, our family and friends feel helpless during our IVF and ask what they can do to be supportive. To ensure that you are not stumped for an answer while being consumed by this process, we have created a list of things your friends and family could, and should, do if they happen to ask for ideas. You might find it helpful to simply photocopy this page and hand it to them!

✦ Please treat me as though I am in a crisis. I am. I can and will cry at the drop of a hat. I am sad, angry, scared, excited, hopeful, worried, and nervous.

✦ Please DO NOT tell me that you know how I feel unless you, yourself, have endured an IVF cycle. This is more difficult on me than you know.

✦ Please treat me with kid gloves, as I am hanging on by a very thin emotional thread.

✦ Please see that everything is not business as usual in my life, household, and heart.

✦ Please call, write, or send me an e-mail.

✦ Please give me books or magazines that I can leave in my car for reading during the endless streams of medical waiting rooms that I will visit over the next month.

✦ Please bake, cook, or order in food for my household. We need to eat and I am out of commission.

✦ Please permit me a clear calendar and excuse my lack of involvement in other activities, as my days are filled with tests, results, endless appointments, phone calls, decisions, physical discomfort, and fatigue.

+ Please offer to go with me to an appointment or even drive me there.

+ Please excuse my lack of interest in everything else. Remember what I said about crisis?

+ Please take my other children for a fun afternoon; they suffer when I am no longer fun.

+ Please give me permission to do what I need to do, be it laugh, cry, sit around, or be really, really active in something.

+ Please help out around my house by washing a few dishes, vacuuming a room, or taking my dog for a walk. Remember that my husband is overwhelmed and in need of support as well!

+ Please let me know that you are supporting me even if the cycle tanks. That is my biggest fear and the hardest thing to talk about.

+ Please remind me that I am strong enough to endure this, as I am sure to forget along the way.

+ Please don't ask me if I am pregnant. If and when that occurs, I will sing it from the highest rooftop.

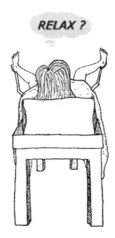

Monitoring Ultrasounds

You will undergo multiple ultrasounds in the 10 to 12 day period of your stimulation phase. These ultrasounds will most likely be scheduled every other day until you are ready for your egg retrieval. Unlike a typical diagnostic ultrasound appointment, the ultrasound tech in a fertility center will give you immediate information regarding your follicular development. It is appropriate to write down the information that you are given. Feel free to ask a lot of questions!

During the exam, information will be collected regarding the number of follicles developing in each ovary and the thickness of the uterine lining. On the ultrasound screen, the ovary looks similar to a block of Swiss cheese with the developing follicles appearing like black holes. Ask your technician to point these out to you. You may have one ovary that is more active than the other. The tech will measure each developing follicle. Usually, only the dominant follicles are measured while the tiny follicles are merely noted in your chart. Pay attention to the size of the dominant follicles. You can ask your tech if the measurements are indicating that the retrieval is on schedule.

Another factor of adequate progress is the thickness of your uterine lining. Many clinics have a minimum value of thickness, which the lining must reach in order to continue with your current cycle. Medication can be given to support the growth of the lining, if indicated. Sufficient uterine lining development is imperative to a successful IVF outcome.

Ultrasounds are an extremely effective, predictive examination and are required throughout the numerous phases of your infertility treatment. Often women are very uncomfortable during the last few days of stimulation. Your ovaries are working hard to create as many healthy eggs as possible. If you have a huge response to the medication, you may experience "kissing ovaries." This is when the ovaries become so swollen with follicles that they touch. This is very uncomfortable, to put it lightly. Your doctor will closely monitor you if this occurs. Tell the tech if the exam is hurting you. You may be able to shift your body position to make yourself more comfortable.

Specialty Pharmacies

All of your IVF medication will be purchased through a specialty pharmacy. Unlike CVS, Walgreen's, or Target, specialty pharmacies carry gonadotropins, injectable hCG, and compounded medications. Compounding is very important if you are taking other vitamins in addition to your prenatals. You can have one pill created that blends several different vitamins and supplements together so that you only have to swallow one pill instead of many. This is a huge breakthrough for women who are being treated for medical issues, such as MTHFR. Many of these pharmacies offer delivery and overnight services. You can request needles, sharps containers, and alcohol swabs. They will instruct you in the proper storage of these medications. It is wise to comparison shop when purchasing your IVF medication. There is a tremendous price fluctuation in this market. Many specialty pharmacies are available online. Ask for several extra needles for injections. For example, the hCG trigger shot Pergnly uses a specific gauge needle. Make certain that you have more than one in the event that you have a flawed needle or it becomes unsterilized during medication draw. Being that time is of the essence with these medications, a delay due to a needle shortage can be a deal breaker.

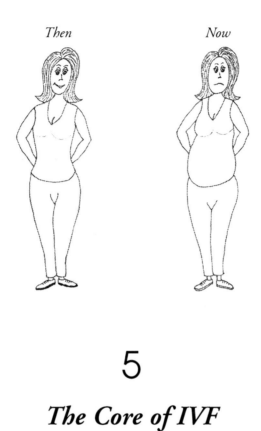

Then   *Now*

5

The Core of IVF

So, by now you get it. A plethora of tests, daily injections, the emotional roller coaster…plainly said, gumdrops and daisies don't factor in to this equation. For many women, neither does adequate comprehension of the technical side of the treatment. This is the beginning of the technical information regarding IVF. Knowledge is power! If you find comfort in knowledge, this chapter is for you. If your inner child just screamed: "Blah, blah, blah!" stick with us, girl! We'll get you through this. The following information is an abbreviated version of a very complex process. Remember, your clinic is the ultimate authority on these topics.

Cycle Basics

There are four primary hormones that play significant roles in a natural cycle, which are manipulated during IVF treatment. The hormones involved are: follicle stimulating hormone (FSH), luteinizing hormone (LH), estrogen (estradiol) and progesterone. FSH stimulates the ovarian follicles. Estrogen encourages the uterine lining to become thick and prepare for an embryo. As estrogen levels increase, it sends a signal to your body to release LH. Ovulation of a mature egg from the follicle is induced by a surge of LH. Progesterone prepares the uterus to accept and nurture the embryo. Human chorionic gonadotropin (hCG) later assumes the responsibility for this function.

Your cycle is divided into three distinct phases: follicular, ovulatory, and luteal. The follicular phase begins on the first day of your period and lasts about 14 days until the LH surge occurs. During this stage, follicles develop in your ovaries. The ovulatory phase begins with an LH surge, which triggers the release of the egg from the follicle. The luteal phase describes the time period that's calculated from the day after ovulation and runs through the remainder of your cycle. Pay attention, there will be a test at the end of this chapter!

Stimulate Me

As you enter the follicular phase of your IVF cycle, your goal is to produce numerous follicles and develop an ample uterine lining in preparation for your egg retrieval and embryo transfer. Many women start the IVF process by taking birth control pills to prevent ovulation and to allow the ovaries to rest. Clinics use this time for a baseline PAP smear, blood work, and injection classes. Depending on your protocol, injectable suppressive medications may begin as early as seven days prior to your next expected period. On approximately cycle day three, your ovaries will be stimulated to generate multiple eggs. Simultaneously, your hormones will be manipulated to develop a thick uterine lining in preparation for embryo implantation. You have been given a schedule of medication that your clinic has tailored specifically for your body. Usually, FSH medications are administered for 10 to12 days during the stimulation phase. Blood and ultrasound appointments will likely be scheduled every other morning for monitoring your cycle progress. You may be required to go more frequently if you are having an exaggerated response to the medication or when egg retrieval is imminent. When your follicles mature, you will enter the ovulation induction phase of your cycle.

Medication Stinks

There are three popular medications used in most IVF protocols. GnRH-agonists (gonadotropin releasing hormone) are used to suppress the LH surge and delay ovulation until the follicles are mature. Lupron is one medication that falls into this category. The side effects of these medications are similar to those experienced during menopause, such as headaches, hot flashes, nausea, or vomiting. Sounds fun, huh?

Follicle stimulating hormones (FSH) are primarily responsible for the stimulation of ovaries. Examples of FSH medications are Gonal-F, Follistim, Repronex, Pergonal, or Bravelle, just to name a few. These injectable fertility drugs are used with IVF to recruit numerous eggs. They are available in two injectable forms: subcutaneous and intramuscular. The method of injection is mandated by the specific medication prescribed by your physician. Do not be surprised if your medication plan changes within the course of treatment. Your body's response to medication is unpredictable. As a result, you may be required to increase or decrease your medication from one day to the next.

The unpleasant side effects of these medications include: bloating, mood swings, tiredness, weight gain, and irritability. Typically, outside of IVF treatment a woman will release one egg per cycle. In IVF, the goal is to stimulate between 10–20 eggs. There is a strong correlation between IVF success rates and the number of eggs retrieved. Stimulation response is the first of several very important hurdles to clear during your cycle.

HCG, known as Ovidrel, Novarel, Profasi, Pregnyl, is used to induce ovulation. This medication will mimic an LH surge, which has been suppressed as a result of the GnRH medication, and triggers ovulation. The medication is delivered through an IM injection approximately 36 hours before your egg retrieval.

Sometimes, there are additional medications prescribed to control the cycle. A few of these might include antibiotics, progesterone, estrogen, and corticosteroids. Know what medications you will be taking, how they are administered, and what their function is.

Approaching Ovulation

Many women are able to tell when they are approaching ovulation. Some experience a distinct feeling of abdominal fullness and bloating that comes from being medically hyper-stimulated. By this stage of the cycle, the countless blood draws and telephone calls for a status report from your doctor have grown old. Every little thing becomes annoying: a bad needle stick resulting in blood on your favorite shirt, not finding a great parking spot, or light traffic on the way to the clinic. By now, you are all dressed up for the big dance and ready to go. It can be shocking how uncomfortable you feel - bloated and sore, like a water balloon ready to explode.

Timing is so important at this stage in the game. You are down to the final few days prior to retrieval. You will be getting a lot of information thrown at you all at once. Be ready with paper and a working pen. There is a lot to document. Know how many follicles look promising. Record the information about their size and which ovary they are developing in. You will be given the date that you and your husband need to be off of work and available for the retrieval. Additionally, you may find it helpful to give the people in your support system advance notice of your big week. Remember what was said about needing a lot of support and help? This is will be the week for that. You may want to fill the car with gas, get some quarters ready for parking meters, and make certain that you have the hCG trigger shot prescription filled. Some doctors specify a certain gauge needle for that injection. Double and triple check your supplies. Ensure that you have everything you need now. When you are close to the trigger shot, clear your calendar. You will be glad that you didn't make plans with your friends during this week.

Many women say that they were surprised at how soon they were ready for retrieval. It can be very unpredictable. If you miss the ideal timing, there is no getting the cycle back. Now is the time to be really involved in your care. Ask a lot of questions. Make sure that you understand the directions that you have been given. If ever there was a time in your IVF cycle to be punctual, this is it. The timing of your hCG trigger injection is paramount to a successful outcome.

HCG Trigger Shot

The last month has been a blur of appointments, blood draws, and ultrasounds. When you have been given the green light to take the hCG shot, remember that the timing of this injection is critical. The hCG trigger shot will allow the eggs to go through a final stage of maturation, loosening the attachment of each egg from the follicle wall that it is growing in.

You may have been given a tentative retrieval date at the start of your cycle. Allow for last minute changes. Follicles can mature overnight! When you are finally ready for egg retrieval, your clinic will call and instruct you on the timing of the hCG shot. After the administration of this medication, your clinic will schedule your egg retrieval as ovulation will occur within 36 hours. When follicles reach 16 to 20mm (1.6 to 2.0 cm) they are considered mature and you may then administer the trigger shot. As a general rule of thumb, follicles over 15mm are more likely to house mature eggs. However, follicles over 22mm may contain poor quality eggs.

Retrieval

The day of your egg retrieval is finally here. You are nervous and may fear that something will go wrong. Maybe the alarm clock won't go off, maybe ovulation will happen prior to retrieval, maybe there aren't any eggs in there after all. In all of the preparation, it is important to keep your focus on the specifics of the procedure. It is imperative that you are at the clinic or hospital on time for your retrieval. You are not going to want to be running late. This is one of the most important days of your treatment. Allow a lot of extra time for travel, finding parking, and getting to the right place for the retrieval. You may want to wear really comfortable clothing. Sweats are a great option as there is nothing binding your stomach. Most hospitals require that you remove all of your jewelry prior to your procedure so it is easier to leave it at home.

Be sure to refrain from eating or drinking anything if you are being sedated. That truly means: DO NOT EAT OR DRINK ANYTHING. (Yes, that includes water!) Coming to the procedure with a full stomach could cancel your cycle. Your doctor or clinic will give you directions involving consumption. Make certain that you follow your doctor's orders exactly as they were given to you.

Once at the hospital or clinic, you will be asked to change into a gown. You may be held in a private waiting room until your procedure. The nursing staff will ask for a medical history, take your blood pressure and may place an IV. If you have not had an IV before, this may be a procedure that you are worried about. Tell the nurse or anesthesiologist that you are nervous. They can explain what they are doing and help you know what to expect. Usually, the anesthesiologist will begin by checking your hands and wrists for a good vein. The selected site may be injected with a numbing agent prior to the insertion of the IV port. There may be some burning and discomfort involved. It is a quick procedure but not pleasant even to non-needle phobes.

Once your IV is placed, you will have some time to sit and wait. Your retrieval and recovery will take several hours. Your husband will need food and a distraction if he is not allowed to be in the procedure with you. He may want to have reading materials, a video game, a crossword puzzle, his laptop computer, or something entertaining while you have the procedure. He may also want to have a charged cell phone and quarters for the vending machine. If your doctor has any prescriptions that he wants you to take following the retrieval, have him write them out and give them to your spouse to be filled while you are in the procedure. You do not want to have to wait at a pharmacy after your retrieval.

Once you are lying on the surgical table, the nursing staff will apply all of the necessary monitors. You may have an oxygen mask to breathe into. Your medical staff will tell you what to expect. Many women find that they get very cold. This is not only a common response to anxiety, but the surgical rooms are often maintained at a colder temperature and you have on a really thin hospital gown. Ask for a blanket. There are no prizes for people who suffer silently!

The anesthesiologist will tell you when you will fall asleep or be sedated. You can request having someone speak to you or hold your hand while you fall asleep. Try to relax your mind and body. It will help you as you are coming out of the anesthesia to be calm and noncombative. When you awaken, you may feel very confused. You will hear voices talking to you but may find it difficult to respond. This is normal as your body comes out of sedation. Do not fight it. You will become alert gradually. If you have any discomfort, tell the nurses around you. When you are alert, you will be wheeled into recovery where nurses will watch to see that you do not develop any complications. Your husband will be brought to you if he is not with you already. You may still be groggy initially. Your doctor will come in to give you a full report of the retrieval. They will know immediately the number of follicles retrieved. However, it will take days to know if fertilization is successful.

When you are ready, you will be discharged to go home and relax. Remember that you may not drive yourself home after the procedure. You will still be groggy from the sedative. You may not feel like going out dancing. Most women report that they are tired and sore for the first day or so post retrieval. Your doctor may give you a prescription for pain medication. Take it if you need it. If you had a high response and many eggs retrieved, you may experience a lot of abdominal discomfort. Lying down, wearing loose fitting clothing, and taking warm baths will help. Don't be obligated into social plans during these days. If someone offers to bring pizza over, take it! You have been through a lot and need some pampering. Your doctor may specify that you should remain on a full bedrest following this procedure. Typically, this means you may get up to use the restroom and that's about it. Be sure to ask what your discharge instructions are. You may experience some mild cramping and spotting after the retrieval. If you feel that it is more than you were told to expect, or if you are in ridiculous pain, call your doctor immediately.

Intracytoplasmic Sperm Insemination (ICSI)

Your doctor may elect to use the ICSI technique for fertilization. ICSI is the process of injecting a single sperm into a mature egg. This procedure is widely used in IVF to maximize the number of fertilized eggs. ICSI allows for couples with sperm motility and density issues or difficulties with egg penetration, as well as folks with unexplained infertility, to move past the fertilization hurdle. Ask your doctor if this intervention will be used during your IVF cycle. Many clinics charge a fee for this procedure. You can investigate the benefits of this in your particular case.

Pre-Implantation Genetic Diagnosis (PGD)

As a result of the chromosomal abnormalities that occur in human embryos, fertile couples have only a 15-20% chance of conception every month. Typically, these abnormal embryos will either fail to implant or result in a first trimester miscarriage. By embryo development day 3, a thriving embryo will typically have 8 cells. With PGD, one or two cells are removed leaving the embryo unharmed. PGD testing allows an embryologist to genetically analyze a single cell from an 8-celled embryo for these abnormalities. Information regarding the genetic composition of an embryo greatly assists the doctor in selecting only genetically normal embryos for transfer, thus giving the couple the best chance for a live birth.

PGD tests for the nine major chromosomes that effect embryo viability. If either member of the couple is a known carrier of diseases such as cystic fibrosis, muscular dystrophy, sickle cell anemia, or Tay-Sachs, the couple may be able to avoid having children with these heartbreaking health issues. PGD may also be recommended for women with a history of three failed IVF cycles or recurrent miscarriages.

PGD is very new in the assisted reproductive world. Insurance coverage is not typically available for this procedure, so you can anticipate several thousand dollars in expenses as a result. There are online resources available for up-to-the-minute information regarding this test. Educate yourself about the procedure and the expected outcomes. Your doctor will be able to help you determine if this may be an intervention that is warranted in your individual case.

Fertilization and Development

You have received information about the eggs recovered. Do not be discouraged if the number is lower than the number of follicles aspirated. This is very normal. Not all follicles will harbor a mature egg. You are looking for the one egg that will make you a great baby!!

Usually 24-48 hours after your retrieval, you are instructed to call the lab for a briefing on your fertilization rate. It is common for that rate to be roughly 60% of the retrieved follicle number. So, if you have 10 eggs retrieved, you may expect to have 6 fertilize. Don't panic if that number is lower than you expected. Remember, it only takes one great embryo. Your lab will give you as much information as they have available. You will be instructed on when to call for an additional update.

Embryo Transfer

Undoubtedly, you have agonized in anticipation of this day since your retrieval. Your clinic has finally scheduled your embryo transfer. This may be on day 3 or day 5 post retrieval. Be sure to arrive promptly at the given appointment time for your transfer. Wear comfy clothes that are easy to get in and out of. Your doctor will talk to you about the embryology report concerning all of your embryos. You and your husband may be given pictures of these to take home with you. The actual procedure is quite quick and uneventful. You will lie on your back with your feet in stirrups. With the aide of a speculum, your doctor will insert a small catheter containing your embryos into your uterus and release them to implant. The catheter will be checked to ensure that the transfer was completed. You will likely stay in a reclined position for up to 30 minutes, or longer, depending on your clinic's preference. You may find it difficult to lie still for the required time after transfer, so bringing an extra pillow to make you more comfortable. Then, as anticli-mactic as it may be, you just go home.

Most women talk about the car ride home and their feelings behind what has just occurred. For many of us, this is the clos-est to being pregnant that we have ever been. Every sneeze, cough, or unexpected jolt, makes us fear that our precious embryos will be jarred from the uterine lining. Yes, it is per-fectly normal to peer into the toilet half expecting to see float-ing embryo. It is nerve-wracking to be finished with the treatment phase of the IVF because there is the lingering ques-tion: "Now what?" You need to follow the recommendations of your clinic regarding post transfer limitations. Now is not the time to become newly active or physically strained.

To avoid feeling as though you may have caused a negative outcome, treat yourself with kid gloves and follow these post-transfer tips:

- No hot tubs, Jacuzzi's or warm baths. Anything that raises your body temperature over 100 degrees is harmful to a potential baby-to-be.

- Nothing should enter the vaginal cavity during this delicate time, including douches, tampons, or penile penetration.

- No orgasms, as they are uterine contractions

- No exercise or heavy lifting

- Avoid all non-prescribed medication, including over-the-counter remedies, without first discussing their use with your doctor.

- Avoid alcohol and caffeine.

Listen, Comprehend, and Prepare

On the day of your transfer, you will discuss with your doctor the number of surviving embryos, their quality, and the appropriate number to transfer. This is a VERY important conversation. Listen to, and repeat back, what you are being told. Do not allow yourself to be caught up in the anxiety or excitement of the moment and miss the vital information regarding the expected outcome of this cycle. Fertilization rates, stage of embryonic development, and embryo quality are factors that indicate the likelihood of cycle success. While you want to hear the best possible news, you need to hear what information is being presented to you.

Understand that your clinic may attempt to transfer any embryo that gives you a chance at pregnancy. Depending on your particular situation, they may even transfer embryos that are not likely to develop, if that is your only chance. This is an important time in the partnership between you and your physician. You need to be willing to ask the tough questions about your chances of success. Is this cycle evolving as your doctor would have hoped? This is a brutal, but necessary, conversation to have.

There is no crystal ball in IVF. A fantastic cycle can fail with no explanation and a poor cycle can result in a miraculous pregnancy. However, there are indications of how hopeful to be during your cycle. Listen for those clues. It will help you and your husband prepare for the outcome.

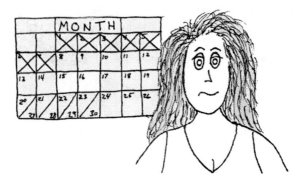

6

And The Survey Says...

Well, girl, you have done everything you can do to make this IVF a success. There ought to be a medal of valor for the prior month of pain and suffering. You should be so proud of yourself for what you have just endured. Ahead of you now is perhaps the most difficult time in this process. You are stuck waiting to know if this treatment cycle worked. There are many approaches to coping with the two-week wait and the ultimate outcome. Give yourself permission to do whatever helps you cope and pass the time more quickly. Before you know it, there will be a definite answer. Either you will be thrilled beyond belief, happy but cautious, or deciding on the next step in your pursuit of having a child.

The Dreaded Two Week Wait

After all of the hubbub of the past few weeks, it is eerie how quiet and long the two-week wait is. There is a distinct feeling that you should be doing something to make this all work. Many doctors suggest that you rest and "take it easy" for the first several days post transfer. Others recommend relaxing and reducing stressful activity for two weeks. You may read lots of different opinions.

"Don't lift anything heavy."

"Strict bedrest for 48 hours then modified activity."

"No baths or sexual activity until after the beta test."

The best advice comes straight from your doctor's mouth. For your own peace of mind, follow that counsel to the "T". It is important to view this time as pivotal to success. Don't do anything that you may agonize over later. The goal here is no regrets. As long as these two weeks may feel, you will be thankful that you did everything within your power to ensure a successful cycle.

It is natural for you to feel tired after you come home from the transfer. You have been emotionally hyped up for weeks. You are bound to feel exhausted and somewhat overwrought. Some women report that they feel pregnant, perhaps for the first time. Keep in mind that progesterone support mimics common symptoms of early pregnancy. You may have also used hCG to prepare for retrieval. This hormone is responsible for many of those symptoms as well. All women are anxious during these days. It is impossible not to obsess about implantation, the possibility of multiples, the thought that the cycle may fail, and all of the other countless worries that creep into your mind at 3 am during a sleepless night. Yes, even the best of us neurotically fretted that our embryos may fall out during a trip to the restroom. It is common to analyze your face and body in the mirror to see if you look pregnant.

In this on-demand society, it seems unbelievable that nearly two weeks must pass before discovering if pregnancy has occurred. For some, it is helpful to get back to work or involved in something other than personal medical stuff. For others, there is nothing more comforting than noticing every ache or new symptom. It is really difficult to know if you should crack out the baby name book and get a head start on the next chapter of life, or if you should practice the "It didn't work…" speech for all of your friends and family. The only way to survive this time is to give yourself permission to do whatever works for you. There is no right way to cope with this kind of stress. It is torture. Period.

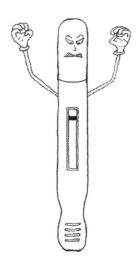

Those Evil Pee-Pee Tests!

Caution: the following information is not for everyone! Some women have the inner strength necessary to defy temptation. If this is you, pat yourself on the back and skip to the next chapter. However, if you simply can't help yourself, here's how to use these tests to your advantage. Before you begin peeing neurotically, educate yourself as to the limitations of home pregnancy tests and when testing is most beneficial.

The use of home pregnancy tests, or HPTs, in an IVF cycle is fraught with controversy. Many doctors adamantly insist their patients resist the temptation of using early home detection methods to predict cycle success. Without question, your scheduled beta hCG tests is the most accurate way to diagnose a pregnancy. The use of home pregnancy tests should never, in any case, be a substitution for that test.

That being said, there are some true benefits to using home pregnancy tests if you are a control freak, obsessively impatient, or just cannot bear to wait the two weeks for your beta test. There are few horrors worse than discovering you are not pregnant via an impersonal phone call from your clinic. That kind of surprise is most unwelcome and difficult to recover from. It also removes the romantic opportunity from announcing to your spouse in a memorable way that you are finally, finally pregnant. Let the Heavens sing!!! For many of us, there is a secret drive to have some control over this medically orchestrated time in our lives. This is your body and you deserve to know what is happening first.

You must be prepared to spend a decent chunk of money on over-the-counter tests, if you choose to monitor yourself this way. The first thing to know is that all HPTs are not created equal. Different brands of tests detects hCG at different sensitivity levels. HPTs can range from 20 ml to 150 ml. HCG levels double every

48 to 72 hours and may be very low in the beginning. Therefore, a lower sensitivity level will be required to detect small amounts of hCG. In the beginning, use the most sensitive tests commercially available. There are tests available that are sensitive to 15-20 ml. The lowest level readily available at your local drug store has a sensitivity of about 25 ml. Most tests are not that sensitive, with the average home pregnancy test coming in around 50 ml. A complete list of pregnancy tests and their individual sensitivities are available on a variety of websites. The FDA requires that individual companies disclose their research regarding sensitivity level and percentage of detected pregnancy hormone at what concentration. Avoid purchasing brands that are surrounded by controversy regarding accuracy and false positives. These brands are a waste of money and have raised the hopes of many women with their evaporation lines, which appear as faint positives.

It may take up to ten days for the hCG trigger shot to leave your system. Simply said, if you test too early, you will pick up the hCG from the injection and will get a false positive result. One way of handing this hCG saturation is to use home pregnancy tests to detect the hCG from the shot on the fifth day after hCG injection. On that day, your test will likely be positive. Continue to test each morning until a negative result is achieved. At that point, the hCG from the trigger shot has left your system. You can now be more confident that any future positive tests indicate an early pregnancy.

Using the earliest home detection tests, you may begin to see a faint positive as early as 6 or 7 days post transfer. Keep testing! Those really, really faint second lines should continue to get darker as you get more days under your belt. Once you have had several positive early detection tests, move up to one that detects a higher concentration of hCG. Some of these tests are fun because they actually have the digital word "Pregnant" come up in the window. This is a great way to tell your husband what is going on. It allows for you to have your big moment without the sterile atmosphere of a phone call from your clinic. Once you get a positive test on a higher concentration home pregnancy test, call your clinic and request a beta blood test. You are pregnant and ready to track your progress via the most accurate methods available.

If you are not finding that the home pregnancy tests are showing even faint positives, do not despair. Purchase a variety of different brands and allow for a little more time to pass. Keep in mind, that not every woman stockpiles hCG in their system in the same way. Many very pregnant women have to wait longer to make a home pregnancy test show a positive result. Although many packages indicate that you can test anytime of the day, first morning urine has the highest concentration of hCG. Do not attempt to drink a ton of water to force urination, as you will dilute your urine and possibly skew the test results.

If you go in for your beta with nothing but negative home pregnancy tests, it is time to start preparing for a failed cycle. Again, this doesn't mean that you are definitely not pregnant, only that you want to emotionally prepare. The goal is to avoid a devastating surprise. Getting a positive beta result after negative HPTs is not unheard of. Be certain to undergo the blood test at your doctor's office regardless of the results of your home pregnancy test. Home pregnancy tests are just one tool to detect early pregnancy. They are not foolproof. Only a blood test will give you a definitive answer.

Beta HCG Blood Test

The best time for a beta hCG is anytime you can get a doctor to allow you to have one!! You were probably given a scheduled date to have your blood drawn roughly 13 days past your retrieval. Make sure to honor that appointment even if you don't *feel* pregnant. It is so important to know what is happening early on. The exception to this rule is if you have had a positive home pregnancy test. Then, you may be welcomed in for a blood test right away!

Contrary to what your grandmother may have told you, there is such a thing as being a little bit pregnant. A positive pregnancy test is not the final answer in the infertility game. There are two types of beta hCG blood tests. The first is a qualitative. This test answers either yes or no, pregnant or not pregnant. This is merely searching for hCG in your blood stream. For the casual reproducer, this test may be appropriate. If you are reading this, there is nothing casual about your fertility!

You are most likely scheduled for a quantative beta hCG. This test measures how much hCG is in your bloodstream with a numerical value. In early pregnancy, this number can be very low. Most clinics consider a value above 25 to indicate pregnancy. Commonly, if your value is less than five, you are not pregnant and did not implant. A value between 5 and 20 may indicate a chemical pregnancy, meaning your embryo implanted but failed to develop. At those levels, many doctors will ask you to remain cautiously optimistic.

Ideally, you want your hCG level to fall within the expected range for your number of days post transfer. You can find these values on a multitude of websites dedicated to the beta hCG test. After you have had a positive beta test, you may be ask to return for a second blood draw with the next few days. Your doctor expects your beta value to double roughly every 48 to 72 hours. If your number does not go up as expected or begins to fall, there are immediate concerns that a miscarriage is imminent. If your numbers are slow to double or don't exhibit a 66%

daily rise, there is a concern of a possible ectopic pregnancy. Tracking your beta values allows your doctor to follow the health of your pregnancy until the 6-week ultrasound documents a beating heart.

When It's Negative

Perhaps you had an inkling that you didn't "feel" pregnant. Maybe you took four hundred home pregnancy tests to be certain. Hopefully, you were not completely unprepared for the news that you are not pregnant from *this* IVF cycle. No matter how you try to work it through your head, it is always devastating to hear that treatment didn't work. The stages of grief rear their ugly heads. How can this be? Why didn't this work? What am I going to do now? It is perfectly appropriate, normal, healthy, and expected to climb on the pity pot and feel horrendously sorry for yourself and your spouse. It isn't fair. There is no explanation on why good, decent, normal, loving people are not blessed with the family that they long for. Many women say that they swing between anger and sadness-devastation and determination. All emotions are fair game. You earned this open season of reflection and contemplation.

For some, there is a need to wrap up all loose ends and jump right back on that wagon. You may want to schedule your next appointment immediately. You could feel ready and interested in your next cycle, or the next stage in treatment be it donor eggs or sperm, adoption or living childfree. Some women feel that they need a time-out from all of the medical intervention. You may need time and space to regroup. It is okay to take either path. Whatever works for you. No one will be able to tell you what is best for you and your partner. You will have to discuss it and think about what feels right.

There are therapists that can help you sort out your choices and help you move forward. RESOLVE has several resources for support in your community. You have friends, family, coworkers, and people in your world who care about you and your disappointment. Now is a good time to call in the support, love, and understanding that you need.

When you are ready, it can be very encouraging to look at the assisted reproductive technology statistics for IVF. Three cycles of IVF is considered the norm for the pregnancy you are hoping to achieve. Your doctor may tell you that there was valuable information gained from your last cycle. Even minute changes in the medication protocol can dramatically change the outcome. If you feel that your relationship with your doctor or clinic has been compromised, you may take this time to get a second or third opinion of your case. Sometimes, a change of clinic feels so much better. It offers a fresh start and a new perspective. Now that you know more about the treatment process and your individual fertility issues, you may be a better consumer of your medical care.

When It's Positive

Perhaps you felt a bit different. Maybe there was a gradual second line on the multitude of HPT's that you had taken. Or, maybe you got a fantastic phone call from your clinic. There is nothing in the world like hearing that you are PREGNANT. Shouldn't there be a national announcement of some kind? The euphoria of knowing that the IVF worked is incomparable to all other emotions. You will always remember this time, where you were, what you were thinking, saying, and doing. If you have not been prone to spontaneous dancing before, you will be now!

You now have to transition your thinking to being pregnant instead of trying to get pregnant. There will be a few follow-up blood tests and the need to continue on progesterone support, based on your doctor's advice. Many infertility clinics will have you schedule an appointment with your OB/GYN by the end of the tenth week of pregnancy. They are dying to cut you loose into the world of mothers-to-be. You are what they work so hard for. The admiration felt is truly mutual. They know how hard you have worked for this pregnancy and are delighted by the joint success.

Although you will no longer be an active patient of your infertility clinic, make sure to stay in touch. They love to get follow up letters and pictures! Strangely, your pregnancy will always feel different than a natural conception. It is, perhaps, just a tiny bit more thrilling, more precious, and more treasured than others. It represents the one time that you can be certain that you have experienced a miracle.

Remaining Embryos

For some women, there is the hope of trying a frozen embryo transfer (FET). During the IVF egg retrieval and fertilization, you may have had more fertilized, healthy embryos than you could transfer. If your clinic matured these embryos and froze them for future cycles, you will have an opportunity to attempt to get pregnant again without the need for stimulation and egg aspiration. The FET cycle is less invasive and less expensive than an IVF cycle. Regardless of the outcome of your cycle, this may be a terrific affair to look forward to.

Conclusion

We can only hope that this book has helped you stay informed and empowered throughout your IVF experience. Not being medical professionals, we attempted to make this complicated topic user-friendly and accurate for all women. Our biggest goal was to assist in the collection of information regarding IVF treatment. Your doctor is the best source of this information. In our own personal journeys with IVF, we established wonderful, close, working relationships with our physicians. We could never thank our doctors enough for their knowledge, care, and kindnesses displayed during the most difficult of times. We are so eager to hear news from our readers who have been successful and to offer our loving support to those who continue to struggle. Keep in touch with us and share your story on our website: www.thewaywardstork.com. We wish you health, success, and loads of baby dust.

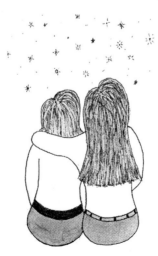

Glossary

Anovulation: A condition that occurs when a woman fails to ovulate.

Antibodies: Naturally occurring chemicals, created by your immune system, to fight infection or attack foreign substances in your body. These antibodies may be responsible for attacking sperm or an embryo resulting in fertility complications.

Antisperm Antibodies: Antibodies that attach to sperm and compromise their ability to fertilize an egg.

Aspiration: The method of extracting your eggs from your ovaries by inserting a needle through your vaginal cavity.

Assisted Hatching: A technique used to puncture the shell surrounding the egg so that the embryo can "break out" and implant in the uterus.

Assisted Reproductive Technology (ART): A catch-all phrase for the procedures that you undergo for the purpose of establishing a pregnancy. ART includes assisted hatching, In Vitro Fertilization (IVF), Frozen Embryos Transfers (FET), Preimplantation Genetic Diagnosis (PGD), and Intracytoplasmic Sperm Injection (ICSI).

Beta hCG Test: The blood test which measures the amount of hCG in your system. Typically an hCG value less than five is considered negative.

Blastocyst: The advanced stage of embryo development just prior to hatching and implantation.

Cervix: The canal that leads from your uterus to your vagina, commonly referred to as the "neck of the uterus."

Corpus Luteum: The yellow tissue that develops from your follicle after it has released a mature egg during ovulation. It produces progesterone, which is responsible for thickening your uterine lining in preparation for the fertilized egg.

Cryopreservation: The process of preserving your embryos for later implantation by freezing them at a very low temperature to keep them viable.

Cumulus Oophorus: The protective layer of cells in a developing follicle, in which the female egg is embedded prior to ovulation.

Donor Eggs: The eggs that are obtained from the ovaries of another woman, which are then fertilized by sperm by your husband's sperm and placed into your uterus during IVF.

Donor Sperm: Sperm collected from a male, other than your husband, which is used in IVF to fertilize the egg.

Egg Retrieval: The minor surgical procedure performed by inserting a needle through the upper vaginal wall, under ultrasound guidance, directly into the ovary to aspirate the fluid and mature egg from each follicle. The hCG trigger shot aides in the release of the mature egg from the wall of the ovarian follicle in preparation for your retrieval. This procedure may also be performed during laparoscopy.

Ejaculation: The release of semen expelled from the testicles through the opening of the penis during a male orgasm.

Embryo: The early products of conception defined as the stages between the first division of cells in a fertilized egg until it becomes a fetus.

Embryo Transfer: The process of placing a fertilized egg into your uterus during IVF.

Endometrium: The layer of tissue, which lines your uterus, that builds up and sheds off in response to hormonal stimulation. The build up of your uterine lining is required to provide adequate nourishment for a developing embryo. If pregnancy does not occur, then this lining is expelled during your period.

Estradiol (E2): The primary estrogen produced by the ovaries. This hormone is responsible for follicular growth and development of the uterine lining.

Estrogen: The group of female sex hormones. (E1, E2, and E3)

Fallopian Tubes: The two long, slender tubes through which the egg travels to the uterus once released from the ovaries when you ovulate.

Fertility Workup: The medical examination and tests performed prior to the start of your IVF cycle, in order to diagnose the probable causes of your infertility.

Fertilization: The penetration of the egg by the sperm resulting inan embryo.

Follicles: The fluid-filled sacs in the ovary, which contains a developing egg. During your IVF cycle, follicles are measured through ultrasound examination until their size indicates egg maturity.

Follicle Stimulating Hormone (FSH): A pituitary hormone that stimulates follicular growth. An elevation in FSH on cycle day three may indicate a reduced egg supply or a compromise of egg quality.

Follicular Phase: The first phase of your menstrual cycle in which follicles grow and the uterine lining thickens. This phase spans between the first day of your period through ovulation.

Gamete: A mature male or female reproductive cell, commonly known as the sperm or egg.

Gonadotropins: Hormones that control reproductive activity including egg production. Follicle stimulating hormone (FSH) and lutenizing Hormone (LH) are both gonadotropins.

Gonadotropin Releasing Hormone (GnRH): A hormone secreted by the hypothalamus, which stimulates the pituitary to secrete LH and FSH.

Human Chorionic Gonadotropin (hCG): The hormone produced in early pregnancy, which aids the corpus luteum in the production of progesterone.

Hysterosalpingogram (HSG): A radiological examination of the female reproductive organs in which a dye is injected into your uterus and fallopian tubes through a catheter passed through your cervix.

Implantation: The embedding of an embryo into the lining of the uterus.

Intracytoplasmic Sperm Injection (ICSI): A micromanipulation procedure where a single sperm is injected into the membrane of an egg to achieve fertilization.

Infertility: The inability of a couple to achieve a pregnancy after one year of unprotected sex.

Luteinizing Hormone (LH): The pituitary hormone that stimulates your ovaries and triggers ovulation.

Luteinizing Hormone Surge (LH SURGE): The rapid rise of luteinizing hormone (LH) that causes release of a mature egg from the follicle. Ovulation will typically occur 24 to 36 hours after your LH surge.

Luteal Phase: This is the last portion of your cycle. This phase spans between post-ovulation through your next period.

Menopause: A condition that occurs when the ovaries run out of eggs.

Microscopic Epididymal Sperm Aspiration (MESA): The procedure used to obtain sperm, through an opening made in the skin of the scrotum, when a man is unable to produce sperm through ejaculation.

Ovarian Hyperstimulation Syndrome (OHSS): A potentially life-threatening side effect of ovarian stimulation that arises when too many follicles develop and hCG is given to release the eggs. OHSS is usually heralded by ultrasound evidence of multiple follicle growth (more than 25 in number), along with rapidly rising plasma estradiol (E2) levels (above 4000pg/ml). Symptoms to report to your doctor include nausea, vomiting, weight gain, pelvic pain, and difficulty breathing.

Ovulation: The release of a mature egg from its follicle.

Ovulation Induction: The stimulation of your ovaries by medication to produce multiple eggs.

Ovum: The medical term for your egg.

Preimplantation Genetic Diagnosis (PGD): A procedure used during IVF to test the embryos for genetic or chromosomal disorders prior to the transfer.

Premature Ovarian Failure: The medical term used to describe early menopause

Reproductive Endocrinologist: A doctor who has received training in Obstetrics and Gynecology, as well as advanced training in the treatment of infertility and hormonal disorders in women.

Semen Analysis: A test that determines the number of your husband's sperm in the semen, whether those sperm are normal, and how well those sperm move around.

Sperm Morphology: The percentage of normally formed sperm in a semen sample.

Sperm Motility: The percentages of the moving sperm in a semen sample.

Twilight Sleep: A light sedation where you will be made reasonably unaware as a result of medication.

Ultrasound: The non-invasive radiological exam that uses sound waves to visualize the female reproductive organs and track the development of follicles during ovulation induction. For the purposes of your IVF, these exams are performed trans-vaginally.

Zygote: The cell resulting after fertilization of the egg by the sperm.

Reference List

American Fertility Association
Formerly American Infertility Association
666 5th Avenue, Suite 278
New York, NY 10103-0004
Support Line (888) 917-3777
www.theafa.org

American Society for Reproductive Medicine
Formerly The American Fertility Society
1209 Montgomery Highway
Birmingham, Alabama 35216-2809
Telephone: (205) 978-5000
asrm@asrm.org
www.asrm.org

CDC: Center for Disease Control and Prevention
CDC/DRH
4770 Buford Highway, NE
MS K-20
Atlanta, GA 30341-3717
Telephone: (770) 488-5200
ccdinfo@cdc.gov
www.cdc.gov/reproductivehealth/ART/index.htm

INCIID: The InterNational Council on Infertility
Dissemination, Inc.
P.O. Box 6836
Arlington, VA 22206
Telephone: (703) 379-9178
inciidinfo@inciid.org
www.inciid.org

Society for Assisted Reproductive Technology (SART)
1209 Montgomery Highway
Birmingham, AL 35216
Telephone: (205) 978-5000 x109
www.sart.org

RESOLVE: The National Infertility Association Since 1974
National Headquarters
7910 Woodmont Avenue, Suite 1350
Bethesda, MD 20814
Telephone: (301) 652-8585
info@resolve.org
www.resolve.org

978-0-595-35784-0
0-595-35784-9

Printed in the United States
65103LVS00001B/238

9 780595 357840